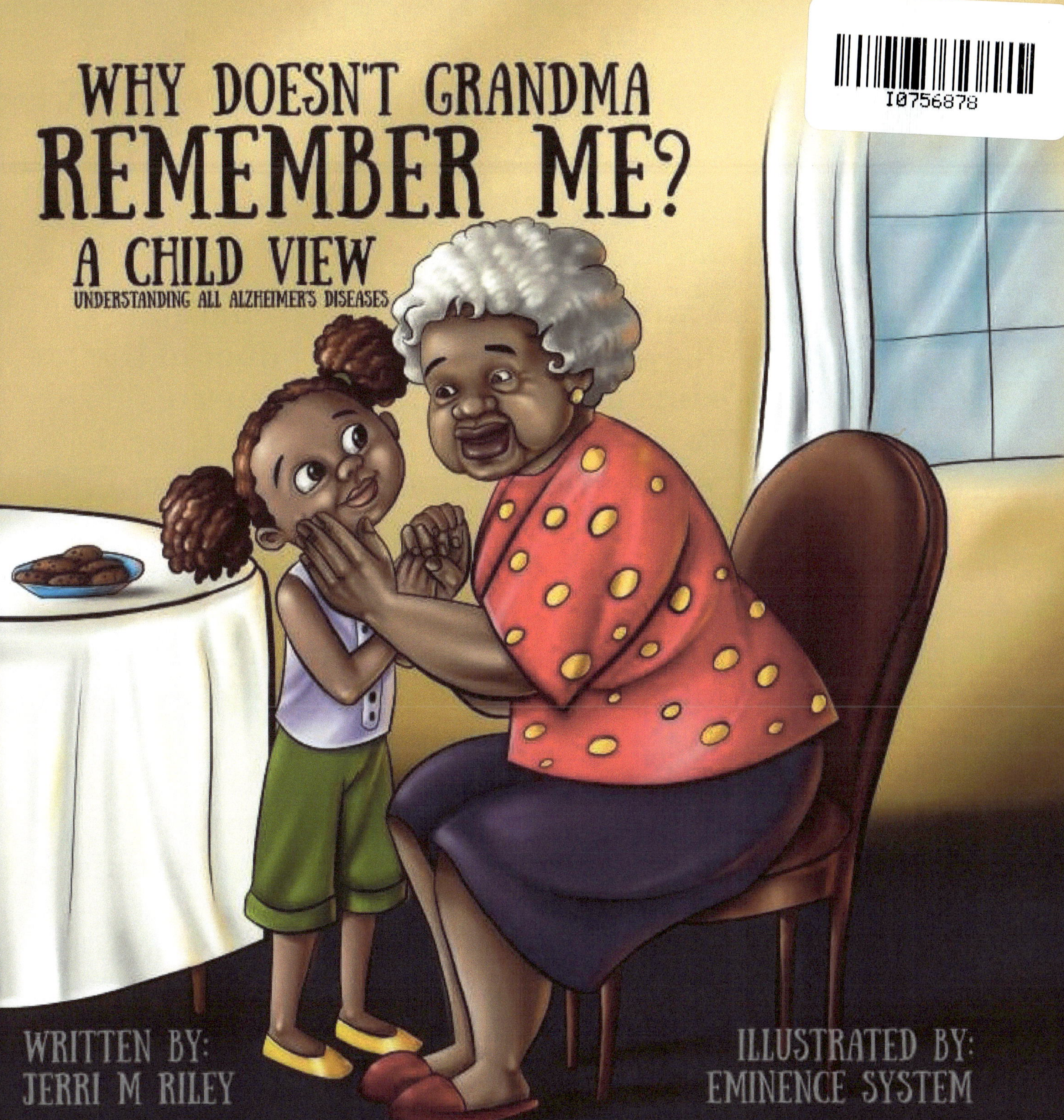
WHY DOESN'T GRANDMA REMEMBER ME?
A CHILD VIEW
UNDERSTANDING ALL ALZHEIMER'S DISEASES
WRITTEN BY:
JERRI M RILEY
ILLUSTRATED BY:
EMINENCE SYSTEM

Dedication

'Why Doesn't Grandma Remember ME!' is dedicated in the memory of Lelia Otelia Blessett-Medford. My mother, who always took care of her family, and made sure we always had what we needed, and also during our family gatherings for holidays and special occasions. You dedicated and spent time with your grandchildren, taking them on family vacations. You traveled on a journey called Alzheimer's disease for 14 years; a long and sometimes, difficult journey that you fought, with all your strength. Your legacy will live on through us and the foundation.

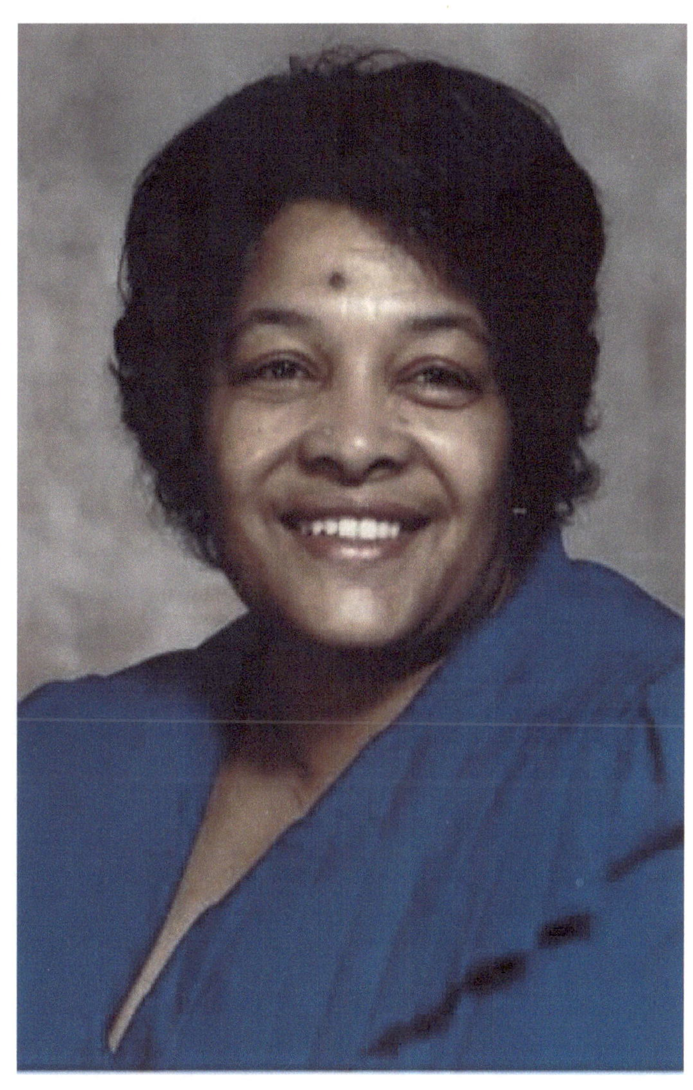

Lelia Otelia Blessett-Medford 2015

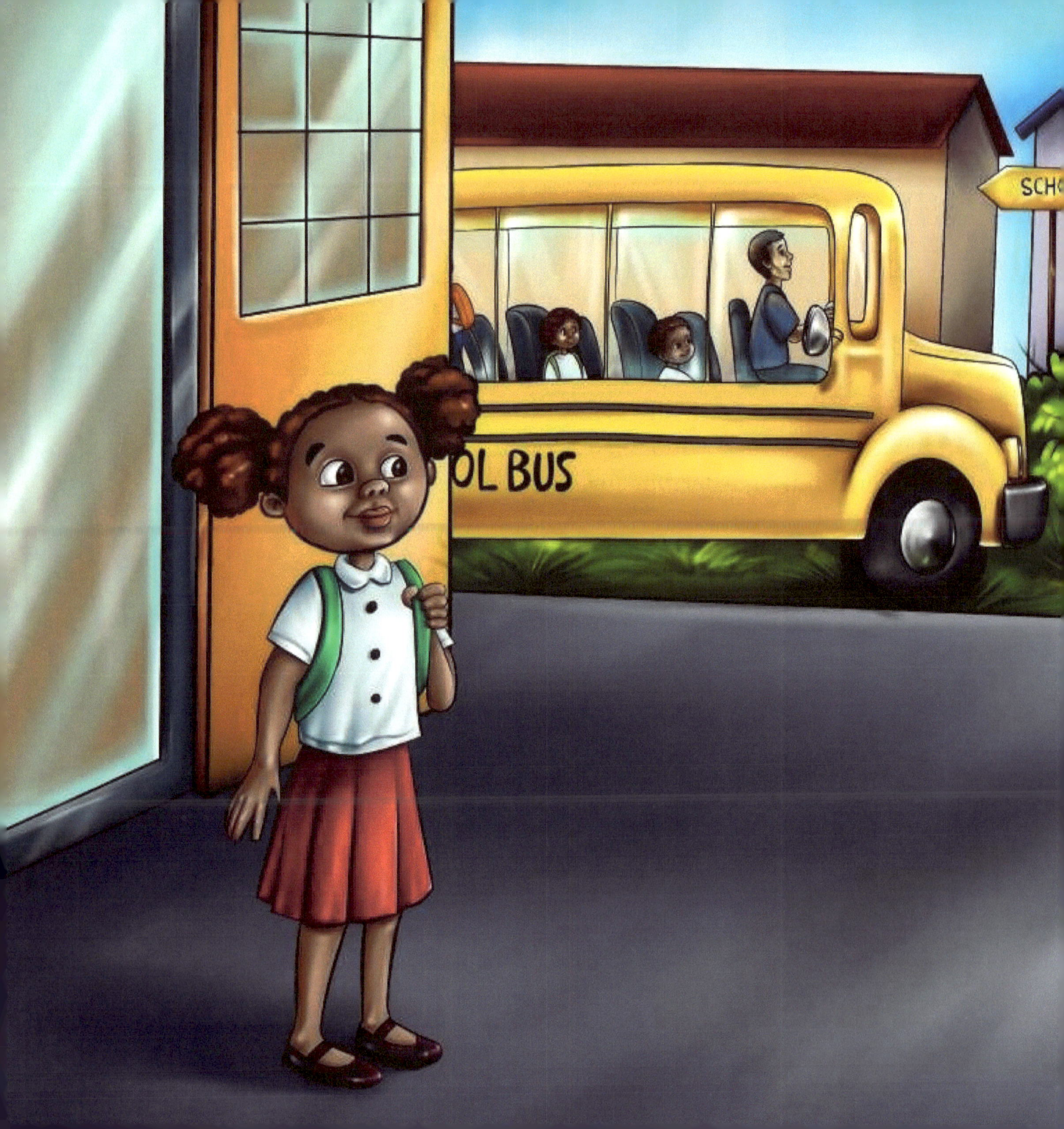
OL BUS
SCHO

My name is Jenna. I'm 7 years old and in the second grade. My favorite subject in school is reading.

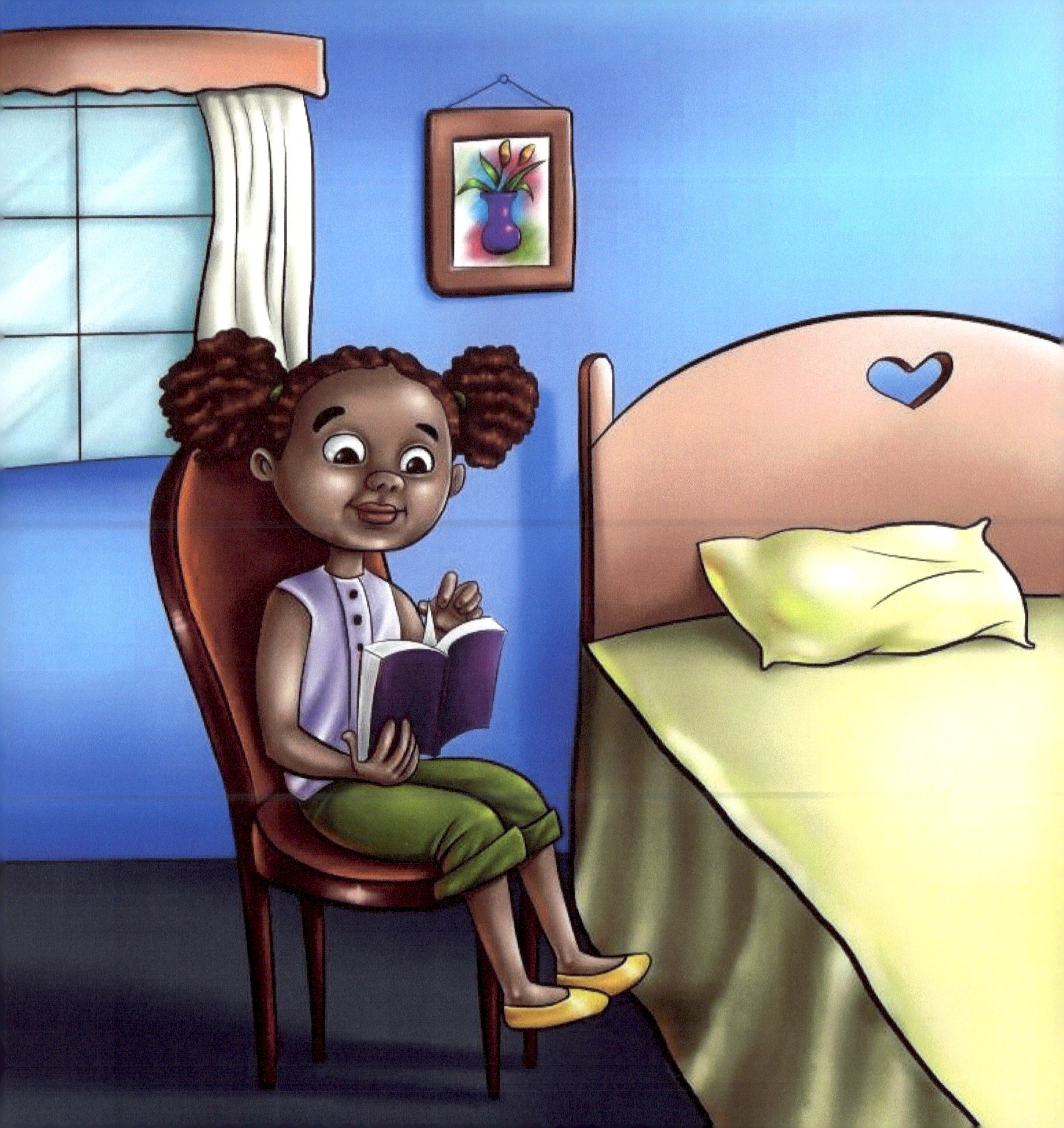

I love to spend time in my room reading one of the many books I have at home.

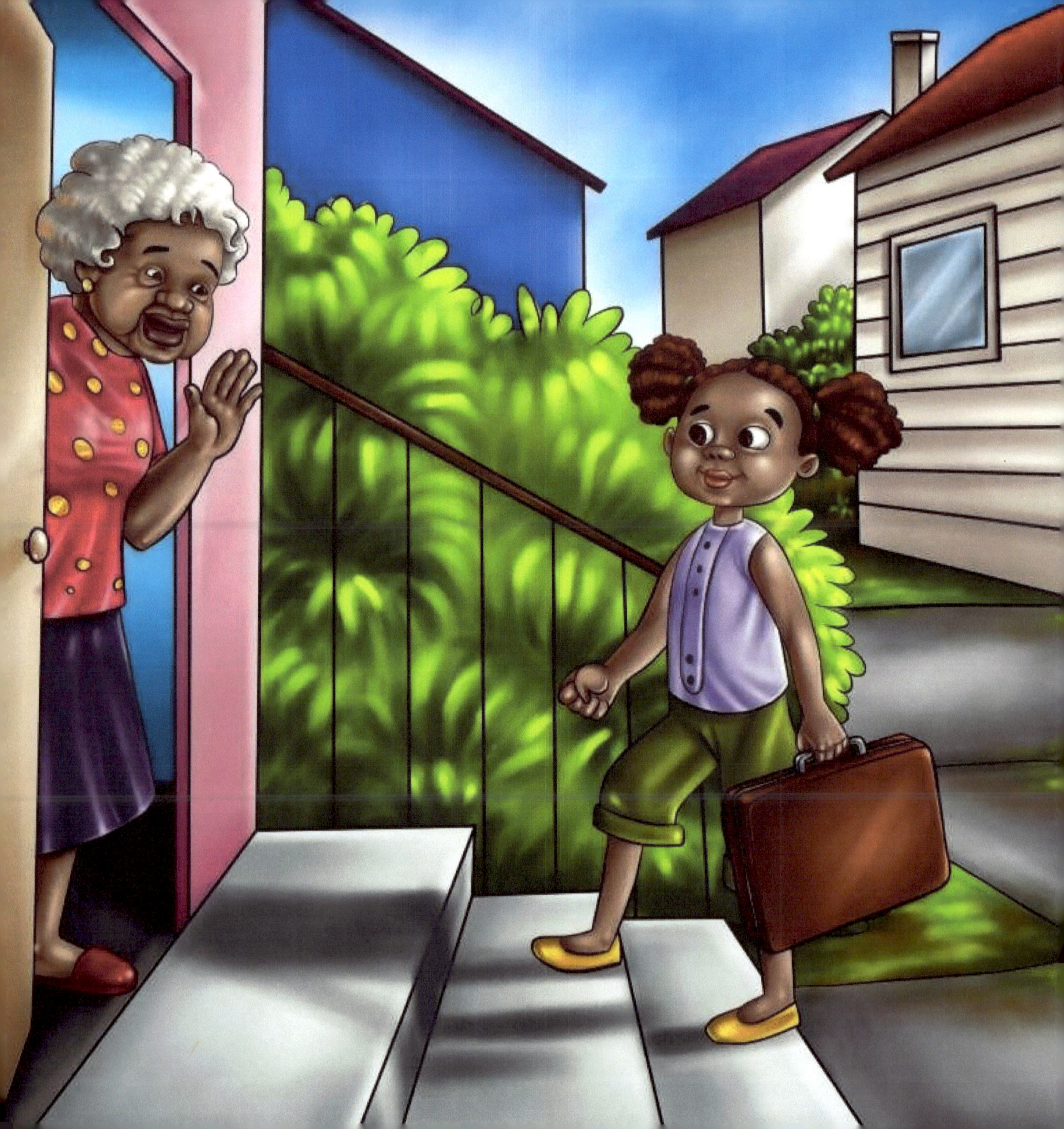

On the weekends and days when there is no school, I like going to visit Grandma and spend time with her. Her house is one of my favorite places to go.

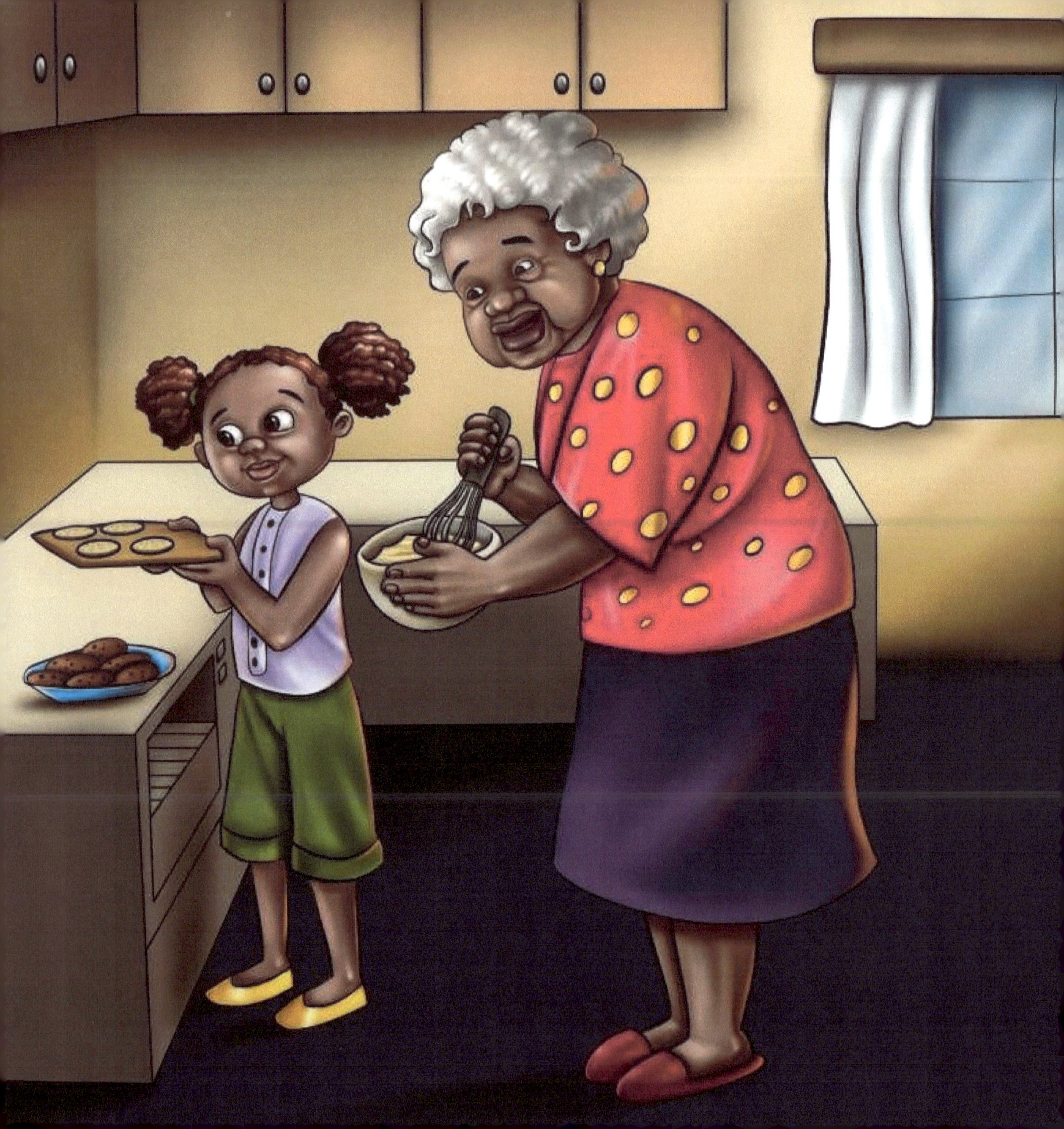

Grandma loves to cook and to bake cookies. We often listen to music and dance. At night time before going to bed, we have story time.

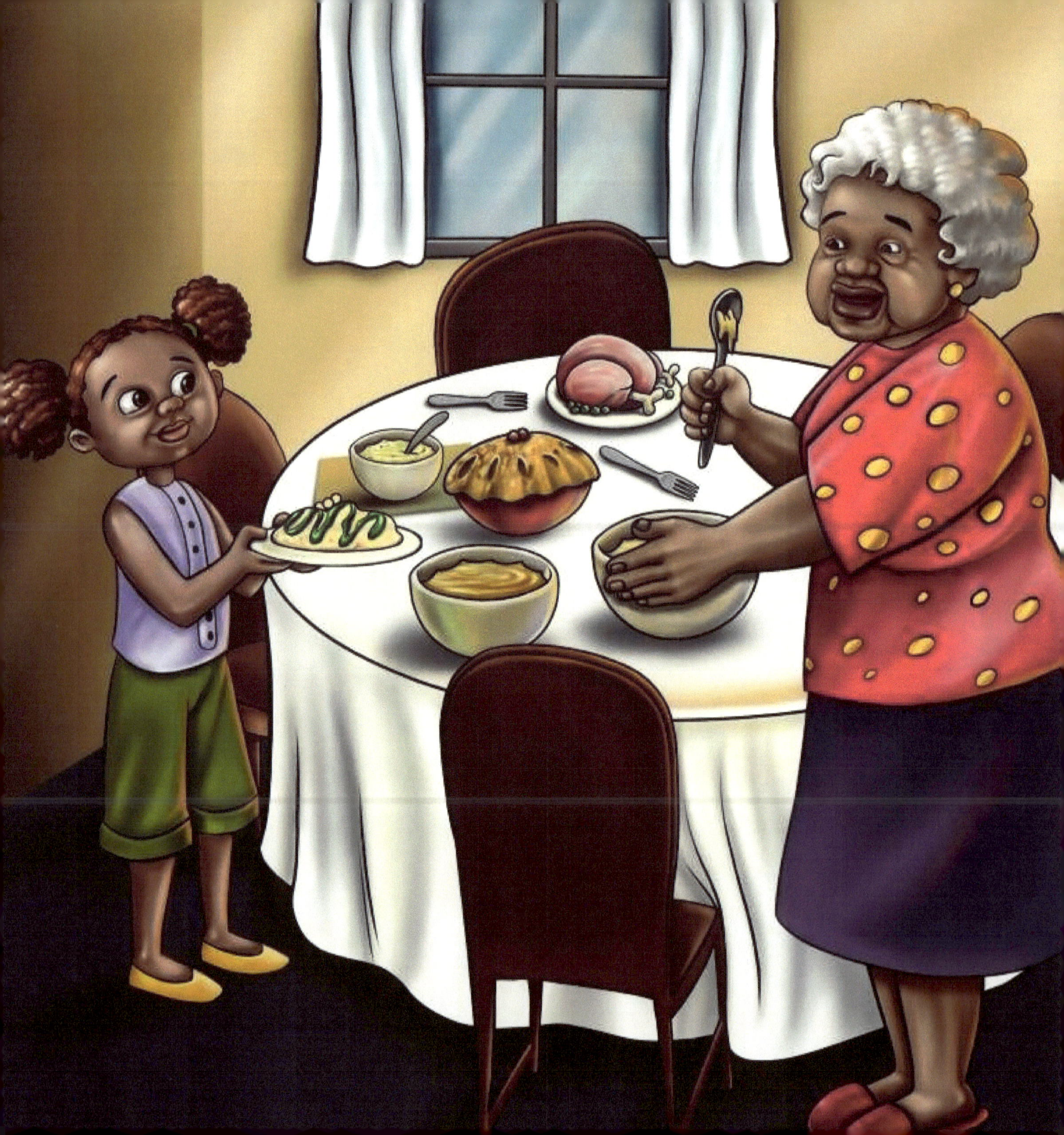

Grandma's house is where we always have Sunday dinners and family holiday gatherings. Those are our family fun times together when we make many memories with Grandma.

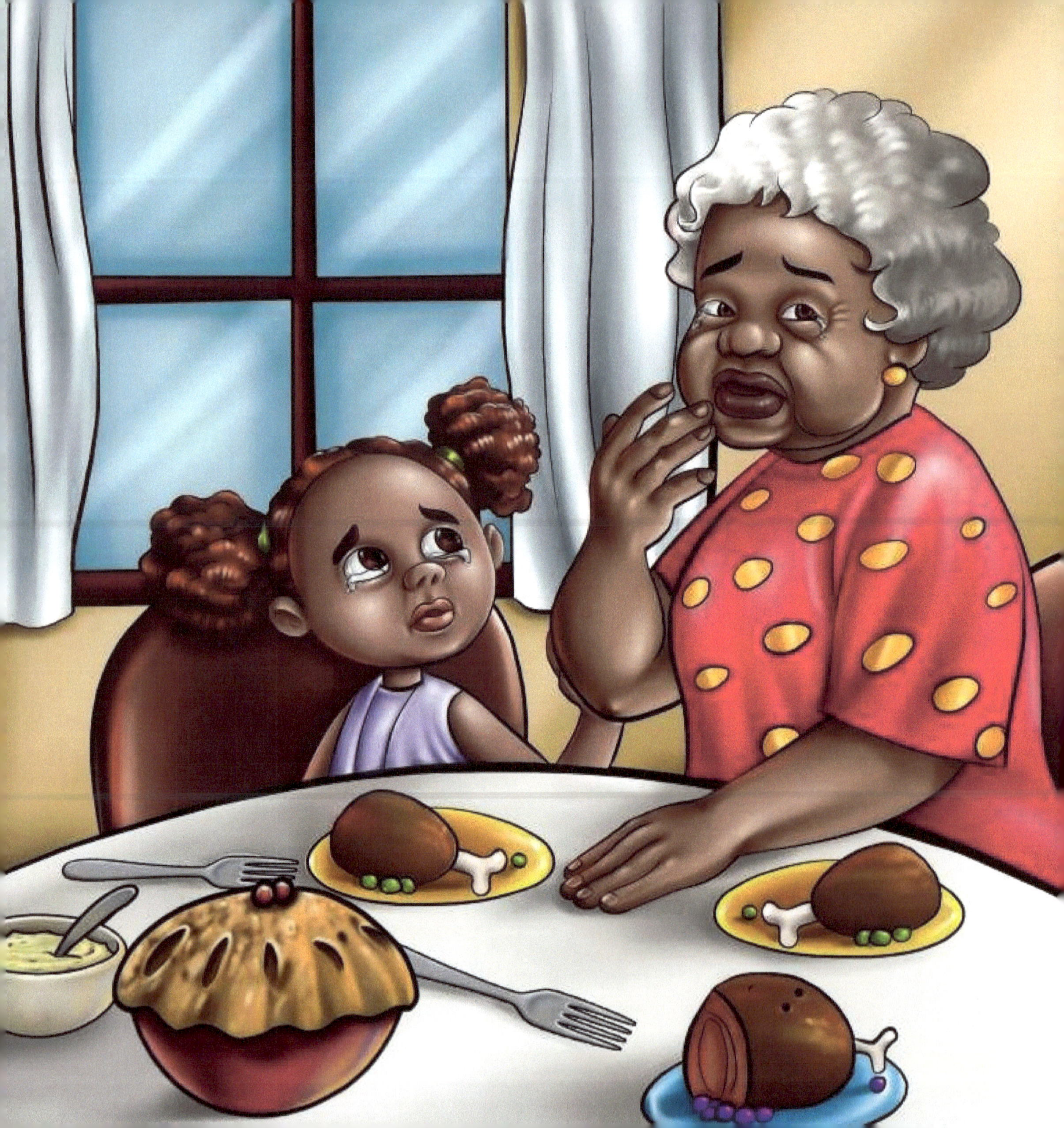

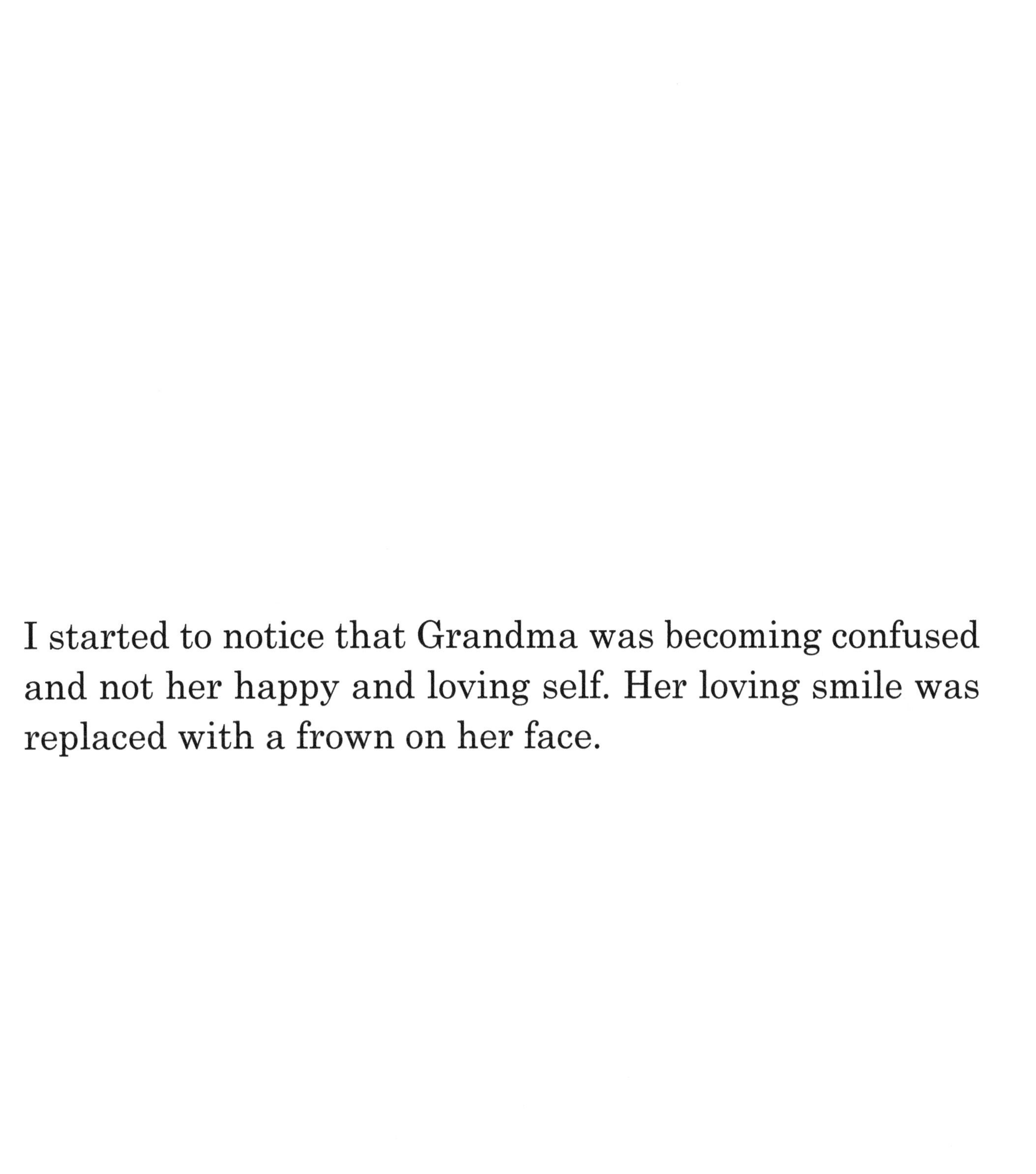

I started to notice that Grandma was becoming confused and not her happy and loving self. Her loving smile was replaced with a frown on her face.

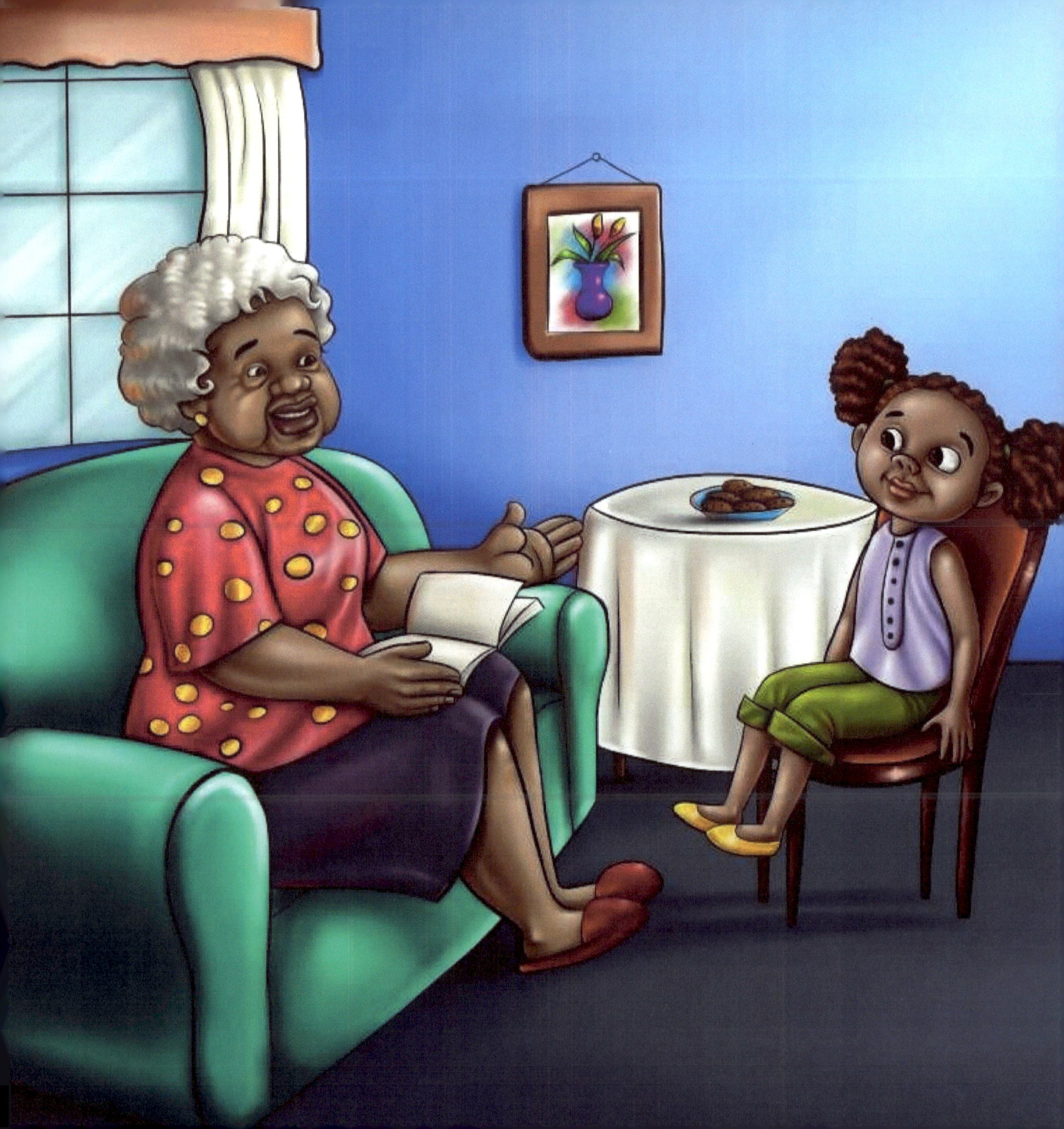

One day I went to see Grandma, and she was very happy to see me. She had a great big smile on her face when she opened the door.
Grandma had started cooking lunch for us, but then she decided we would sit down and have story time. As Grandma continue to read to me, the smoke alarm went off in the kitchen.

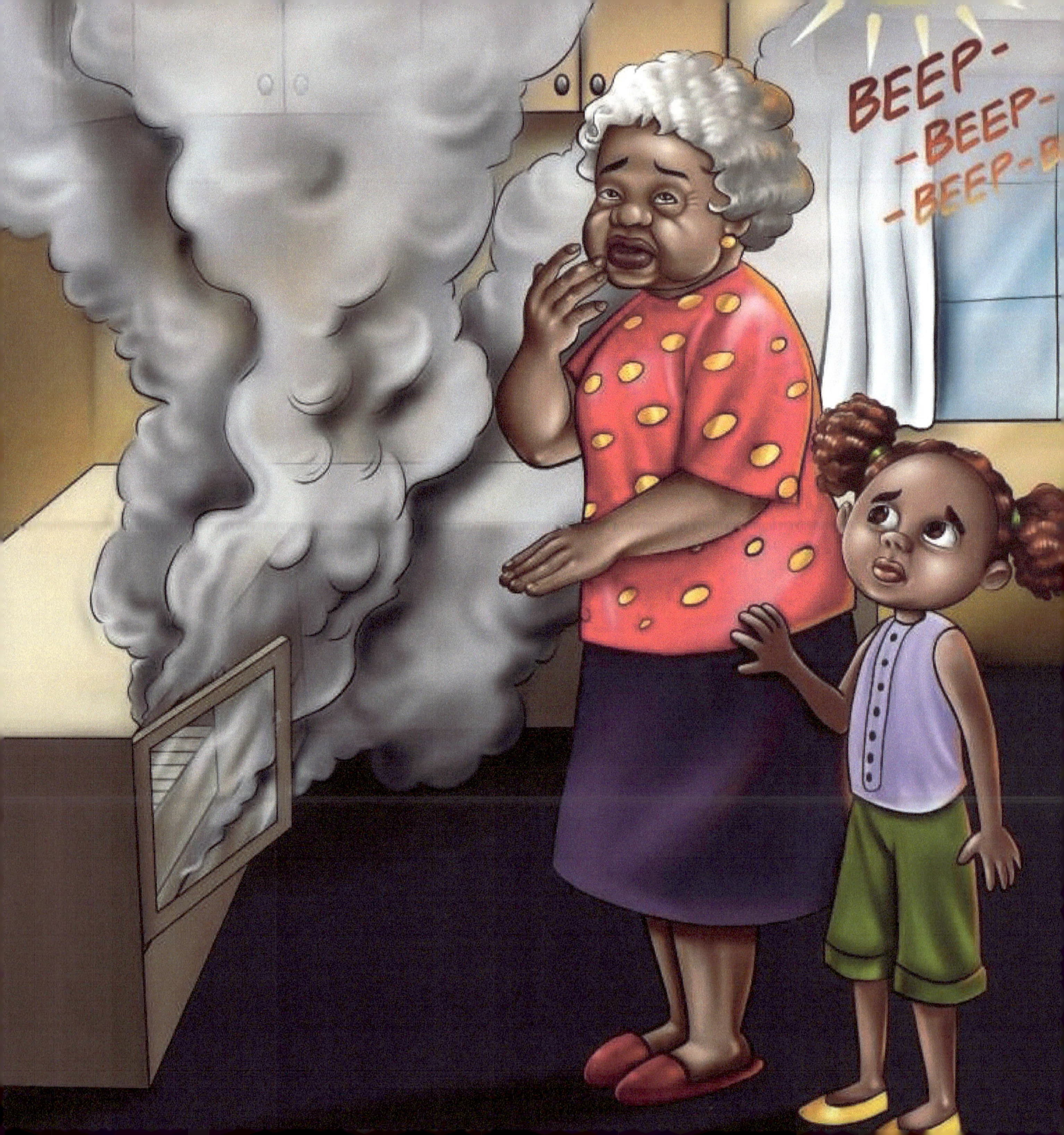

BEEP-
-BEEP-
-BEEP-B

The house filled up with smoke. Grandma became confused about what was going on. I told Grandma the food in the oven was burning. Grandma said, "What food? I'm not cooking any food." That's when I really wondered what was wrong with Grandma.
I told my mother that Grandma was acting different and starting to forget things.

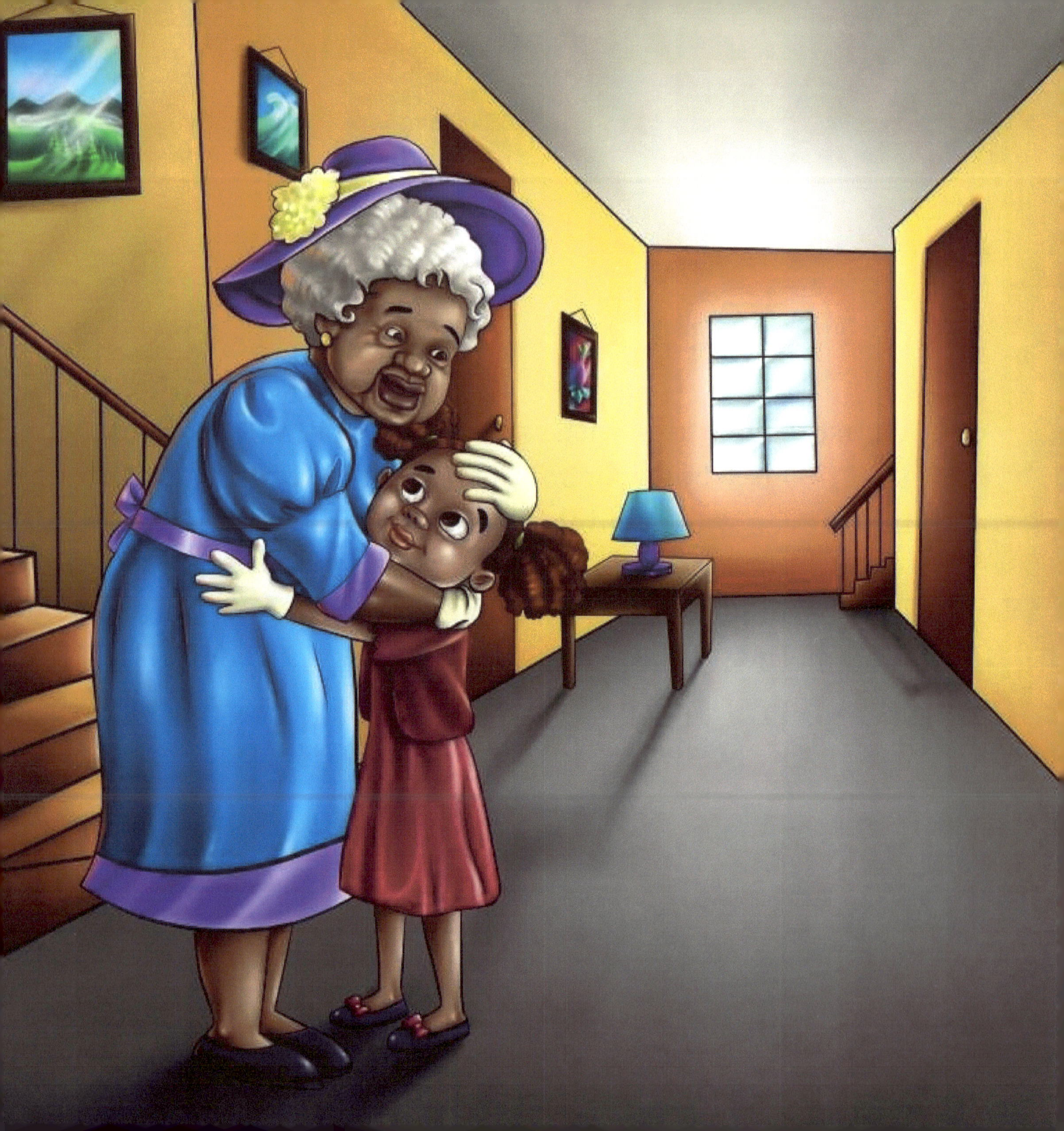

One Sunday after church, we went to Grandma's house to have our Sunday family dinner. I was so excited to see Grandma that day. Mother rang the doorbell and Grandma opened the door.

I gave Grandma a big hug and told her I was happy to see her. Grandma looked surprise to see me and Mother. Grandma asked why we were at her house. Mother replied, " Remember, you wanted to see Jenna today so you could bake cookies with her."

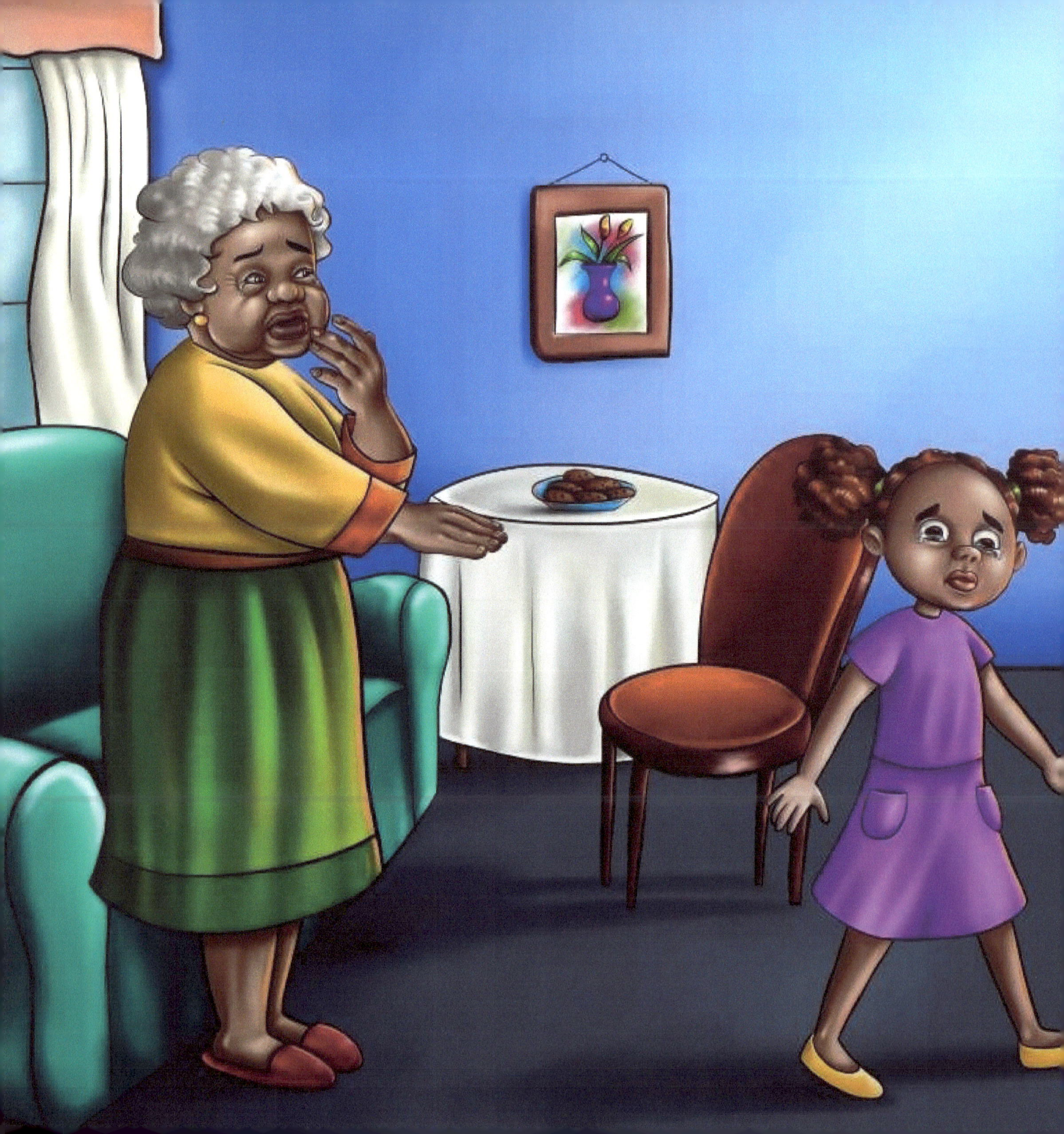

Grandma replied, "Who is Jenna?"

Mother said to Grandma, "This is your granddaughter Jenna."

Grandma said, "I don't know this little girl." She walked away from the door to go back inside the house.

I started to cry and asked Mother, "Why doesn't Grandma remember me?

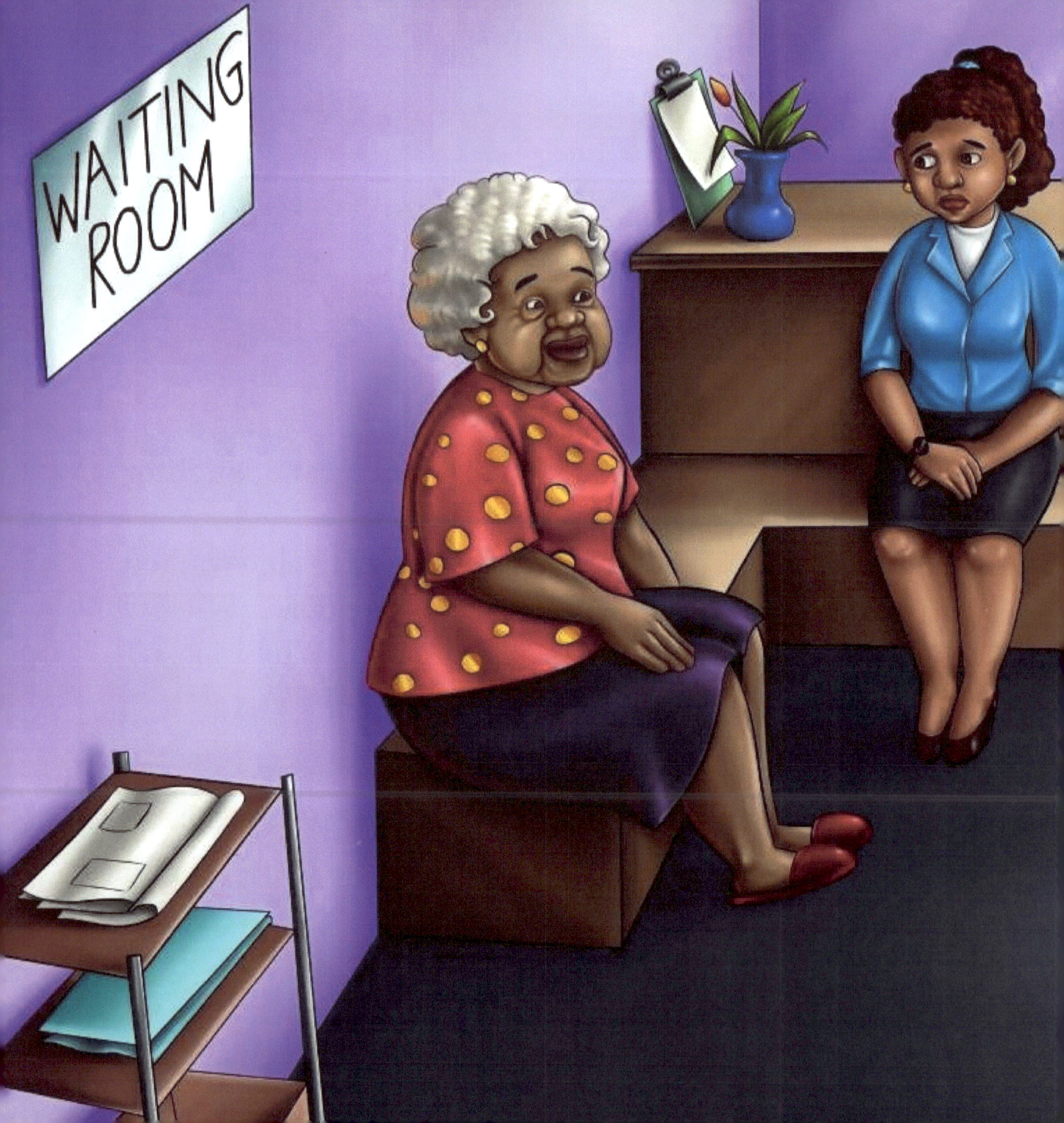

WAITING
ROOM

A week later, Grandma had several doctor appointments that Mother had to take her to. Grandma was not feeling well and said she didn't feel like her normal self anymore.

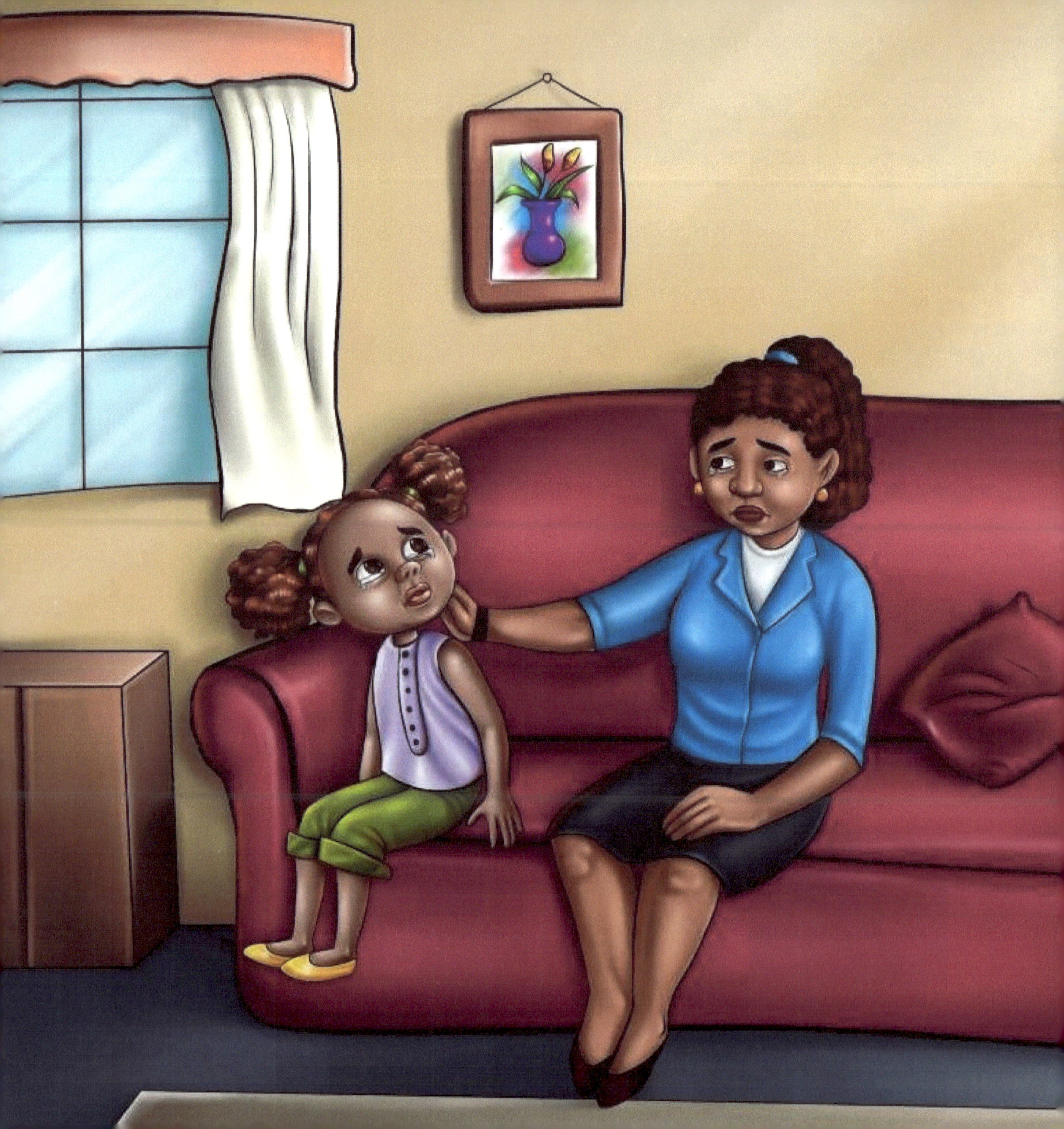

One day, when I came home from school, mother was waiting for me at home. Mother said, "Jenna, I want to talk to you about something."
I could see in Mother's eyes that she had been crying. I asked Mother, "Is this about Grandma?" and she replied yes.

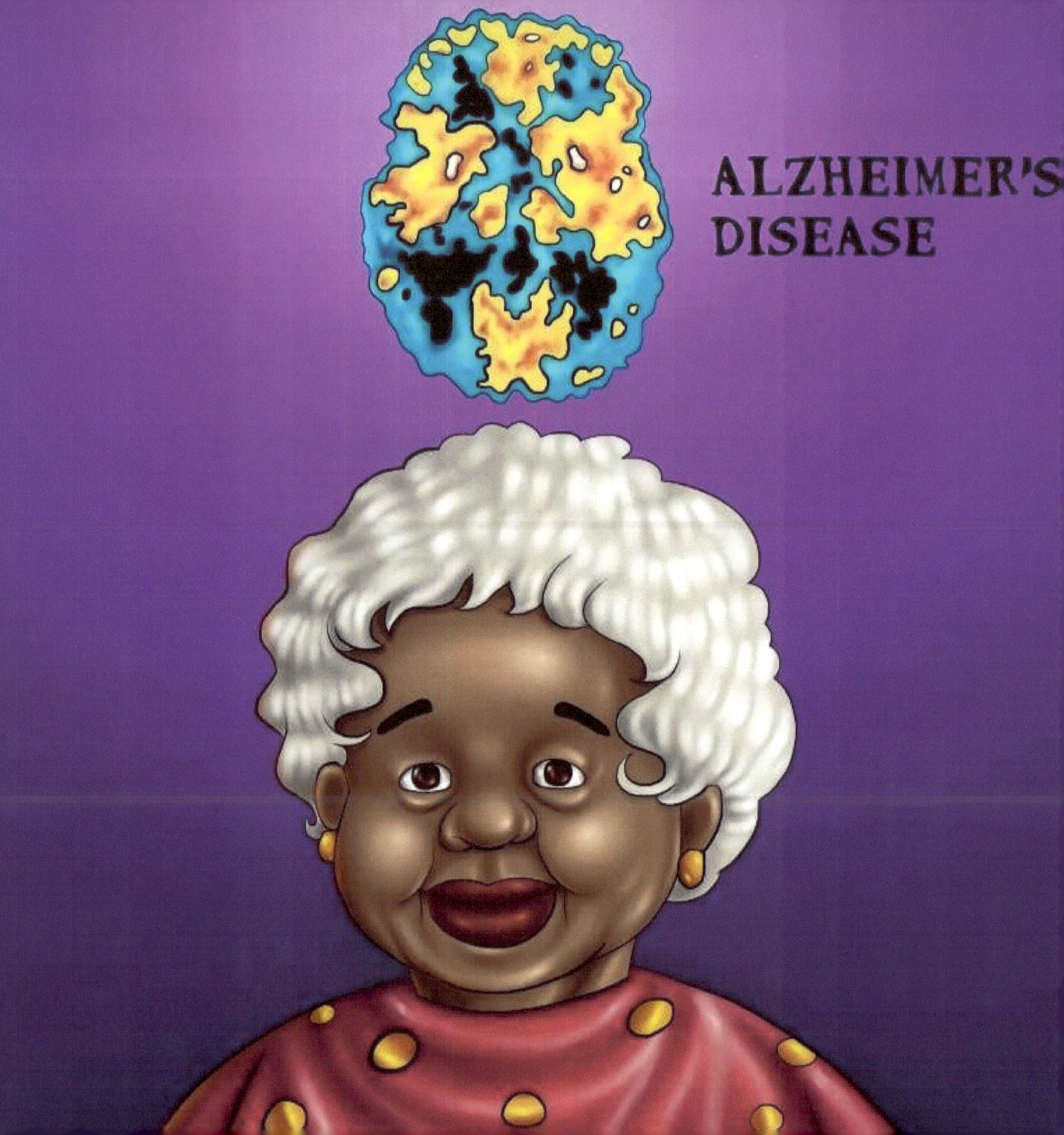

ALZHEIMER'S
DISEASE

Mother explained that Grandma had some pictures taken of her brain and they showed that Grandma had a disease called Alzheimer's. This disease would cause Grandma to act differently and to forget somethings. Grandma would look the same on the outside, but on the inside, Grandma's brain was changing, which would affect Grandma's memory and her everyday activities. My mother said a time will come when Grandma won't remember our names or faces because her brain is sick. There is research being conducted to find a cure for this disease. I cried and asked Mother why this was happening to Grandma.

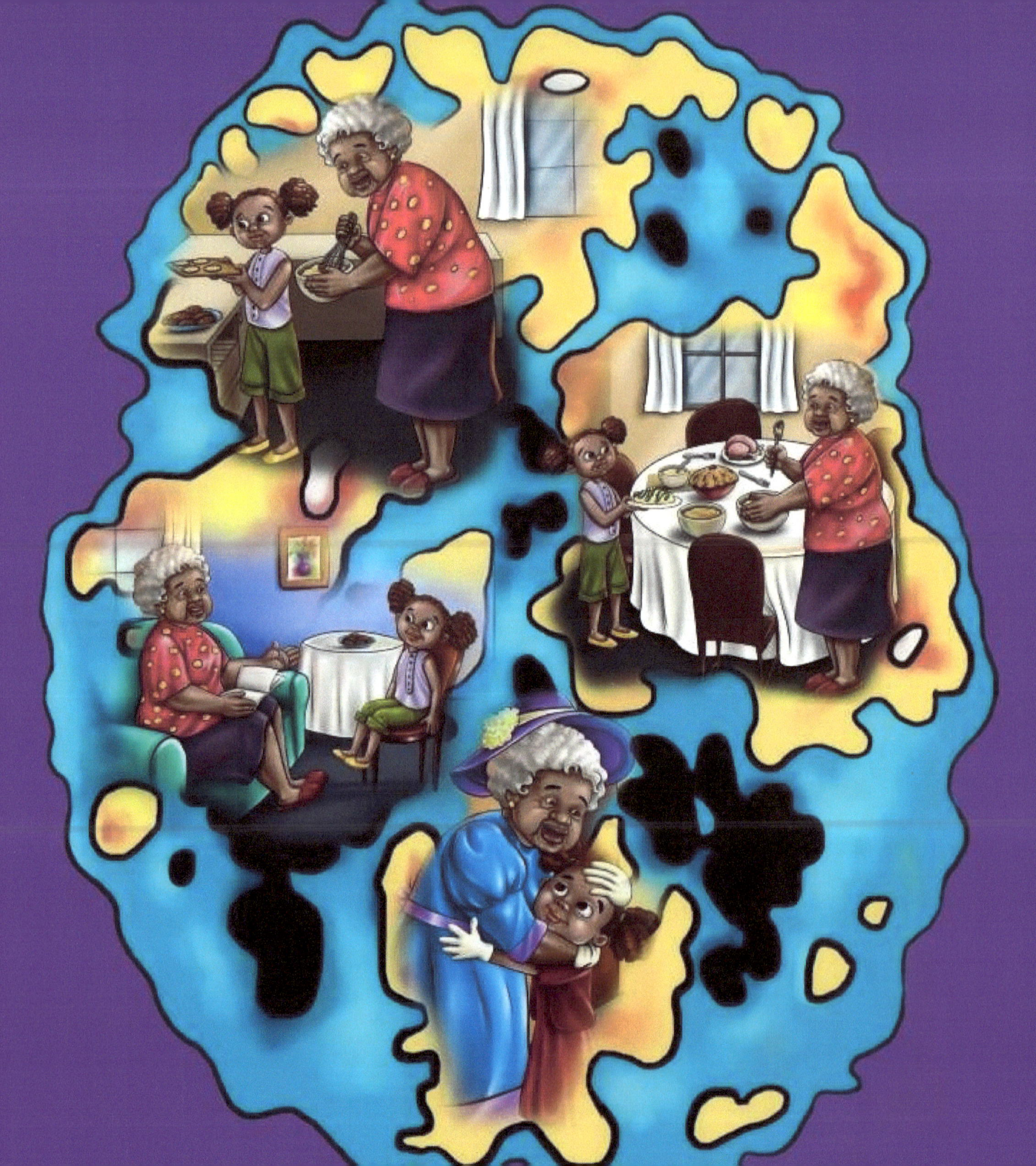

I went to go see Grandma. She opened the door and gave me a hug with a big smile on her face. She said, "Come in, Jenna. I'm so happy you came to see me today." We hugged each other and smiled, and we went in the kitchen to bake some cookies.

Grandma told me how much she loves me and how she enjoys my visits with her. I know Grandma's brain is sick, and a time will come when Grandma will come to live with us, and we will take care of Grandma. A day will come when Grandma won't remember me. I will be there to help take care of Grandma when that time comes. I know I will always be in her heart. I love my grandma!

2018 ALZHEIMER'S DISEASE FACTS AND FIGURES

ALZHEIMER'S DISEASE IS THE

6TH leading cause of death in the United States

16.1 MILLION AMERICANS provide unpaid care for people with Alzheimer's or other dementias

These caregivers provided an estimated **18.4 BILLION HOURS** of care valued at over **$232 BILLION**

Between 2000 and 2015 deaths from heart disease have decreased

11% 

while deaths from Alzheimer's disease have increased

 **123%**

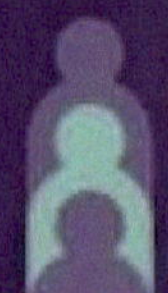

1 IN 3 seniors dies with Alzheimer's or another dementia

It kills more than breast cancer and prostate cancer **COMBINED**

EARLY AND ACCURATE DIAGNOSIS COULD **SAVE** UP TO

$7.9 TRILLION in medical and care costs

IN 2018, Alzheimer's and other dementias will cost the nation **$277 BILLION**

BY 2050, these costs could rise as high as **$1.1 TRILLION**

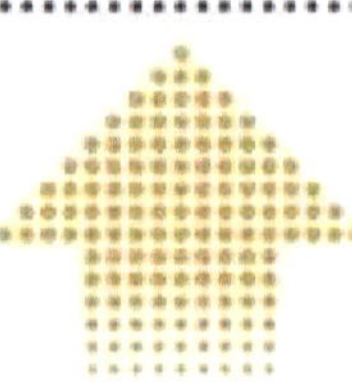

5.7 MILLION Americans are living with Alzheimer's

BY 2050, this number is projected to rise to nearly

14 MILLION

EVERY 65 SECONDS someone in the United States develops the disease

alzheimer's association®

THE BRAINS BEHIND SAVING YOURS℠

10 WAYS TO **LOVE YOUR BRAIN**

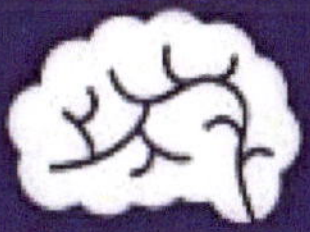

START NOW. It's never too late or too early to incorporate healthy habits.

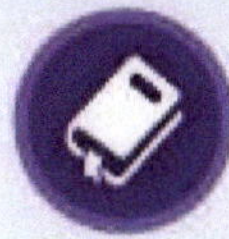

HIT THE BOOKS
Formal education will help reduce risk of cognitive decline and dementia. Take a class at a local college, community center or online.

BUTT OUT
Smoking increases risk of cognitive decline. Quitting smoking can reduce risk to levels comparable to those who have not smoked.

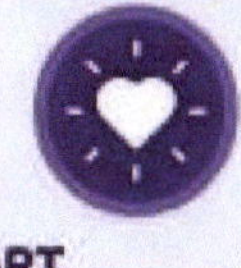

FOLLOW YOUR HEART
Risk factors for cardiovascular disease and stroke — obesity, high blood pressure and diabetes — negatively impact your cognitive health.

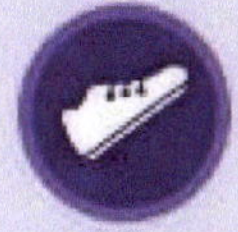

BREAK A SWEAT
Engage in regular cardiovascular exercise that elevates heart rate and increases blood flow. Studies have found that physical activity reduces risk of cognitive decline.

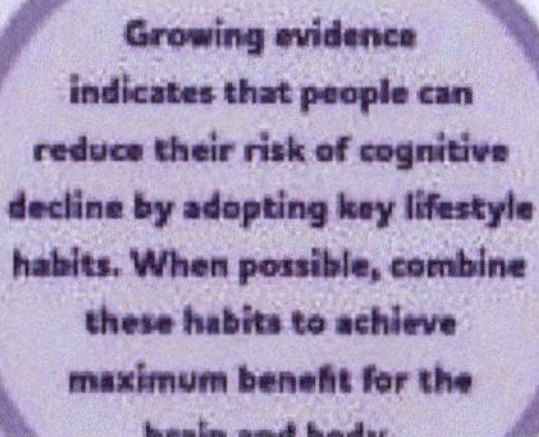

STUMP YOURSELF
Challenge your mind. Build a piece of furniture. Play games of strategy, like bridge.

HEADS UP!
Brain injury can raise risk of cognitive decline and dementia. Wear a seat belt and use a helmet when playing contact sports or riding a bike.

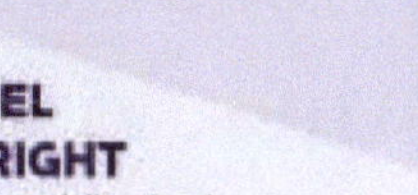

BUDDY UP
Staying socially engaged may support brain health. Find ways to be part of your local community or share activities with friends and family.

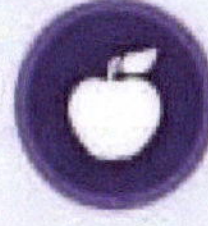

FUEL UP RIGHT
Eat a balanced diet that is higher in vegetables and fruit to help reduce the risk of cognitive decline.

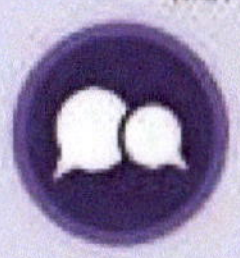

TAKE CARE OF YOUR MENTAL HEALTH
Some studies link depression with cognitive decline, so seek treatment if you have depression, anxiety or stress.

CATCH SOME ZZZ'S
Not getting enough sleep may result in problems with memory and thinking.

Visit alz.org/10ways to learn more.

alzheimer's association

THE BRAINS BEHIND SAVING YOURS.

Alzheimer's Disease defined for kids…
A brain disease of later life that is characterized by changes in brain tissue with gradual loss of memory and mental abilities.

Dementia Disease defined for kids…
A condition of the brain that is marked especially by a deterioration in the ability to think, reason, or remember. A condition of deteriorating mental functioning.

A WORD FROM THE AUTHOR...

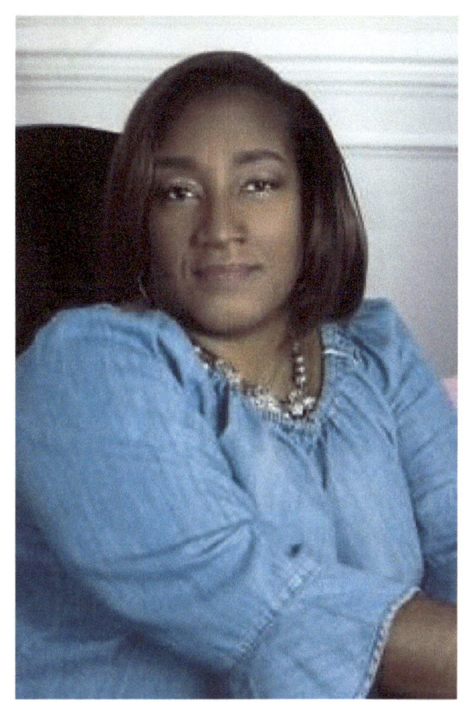

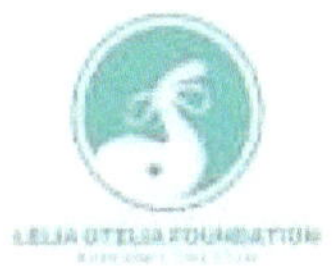

LELIA OTELIA FOUNDATION

Jerri Riley
CEO/FOUNDER

www.leliaoteliafoundation.org
lofound@leliaoteliafoundation.org
256 368 6350
P.O. Box 650
Odessa DE 19730

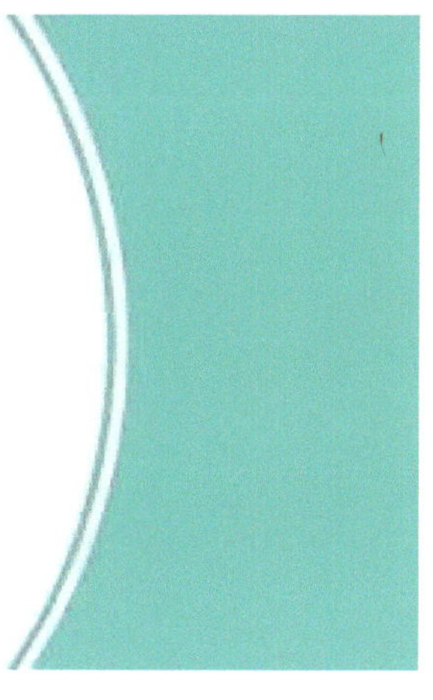

My name is Jerri M. Riley. I'm the author of "Why Doesn't Grandma Remember ME?" I decided to write this book from my personal experience with my mother, who traveled this journey for 14 years. Once an Alzheimer's Disease diagnosis is made, every family member connected to that person, no matter what relationship they have, will be affected by this disease. I chose to write my story with the youngest family members in mind. Our children look up to the matriarch and patriarch of our families. They don't understand when our loved one's behavior change due to Alzheimer's Disease. I believe this book will be a conversation starter, and will help answer questions many have wondered. My goal and hope is that, this book will go into the homes of families, with a passion for educating even the youngest family member about a disease that is affecting our loved ones. Studies and research has shown a younger onset of Alzheimer's Disease that will affect our younger generations in the nearest future.